RoelsMethod™

NeuroSomatic Reset

Mini Book

Chapter One

The Crisis That Changes Everything

When the car hit, it didn't just twist metal—it twisted the trajectory of my entire life.

I was twenty-one, a summer lifeguard on the way to the neighborhood pool for my morning shift. No clinic, no treatment room, no years of body-work expertise—just a young guy riding shotgun, music on the radio, sun barely over the Denver skyline. One moment we were coasting toward a traffic light; the next, a Cadillac pulled across our lane, and the world detonated in glass and steel.

That impact ripped through more than bone and muscle. It shattered the illusion that pain was something that happened to other people. In an instant, I went from a carefree bystander to an unwilling protagonist in a story of relentless, unexplained agony. I wasn't a therapist yet; I was the patient every future therapist version of me would try to understand. And the pain that followed wasn't just physical. It was disorienting, identity-shaking—the kind of hurt that makes you question who you are and why you're here.

That wreck didn't take my life, but it rewrote it, setting the stage for the method you're holding in your hands

My identity shattered right along with my body.

I tried everything: physical therapy, chiropractic care, acupuncture, injections, and countless massage sessions. I followed the rules. I stayed consistent. I did the homework. And yet, the pain persisted. It moved, it changed, it tricked me into thinking I was better—then it came roaring back.

It was like playing a game I could never win.

However, that game is precisely what is being played out in chronic pain care worldwide. Systems are set up to keep people dependent, quiet, and paying. And when you don't get better, it's somehow *your fault*. You must be doing it wrong. You must not want it enough. You must be weak, or anxious, or out of alignment—again.

That cycle? I've lived it. But I didn't stop there.

I decided that if no method could help me, I would create one.

RoelsMethod™ NeuroSomatic Reset was born not out of theory, but out of necessity. It's a system developed to disrupt pain patterns at their trustworthy source, rather than where pain is felt. Still, its origin lies in the neuromuscular confusion and protective compensation patterns that the body creates after trauma or prolonged strain. It's rooted in the knowledge that pain isn't random, and healing doesn't have to be long or mysterious.

Today, I live pain-free, but my return to the world began far from a treatment room. After I was told I would most likely never get better and should just go on disability and learn to "manage" the pain, I began the healing experience that I realized would have to involve my mind and spirit as well as my body. It was either that or give up entirely. Two weeks later, I took a job behind the counter at a neighborhood soda shop and was promoted to manager almost immediately. Stocking coolers, scooping ice cream, wiping tables, and running the place proved, hour by hour, that my body was truly free again. Eight months later, on August 25, 2001—exactly four years to the day after the crash—I enrolled in massage school, carrying a mission that had crystallized in those long, fizzy shifts: I won't just massage; I will reset. I will educate. I will challenge the industry's comfortable dysfunction. And I will help people find lasting relief, often in only three focused sessions.

This book isn't only my story. It's a spotlight on broken systems, a compass for anyone lost in the medical maze, and a map toward a better future.

Pain doesn't have to be forever.
This is where the reset begins.

Chapter Two

How the Pain Industry Profits from Prolonged Suffering

Let's be honest: pain is profitable.

Billions of dollars are generated every year from physical therapy packages, chiropractic adjustments, injections, supplements, gadgets, surgeries, and pharmaceuticals. These approaches are rarely about resolution—they're about *management*. And management means **you keep coming back**.

When you heal in three sessions, you disrupt an entire business model.

I've had multiple licensed professionals —chiropractors, physical therapists, and even massage therapists—say it to my face: "If I fixed them that fast, I'd be out of business." They're not being cruel. They're protecting a structure built on chronicity. They sell extended treatment plans. They rely on insurance reimbursements. They count on your continued suffering. It's a fear-based and codependent relationship, enabling people to believe "one day the pain will stop coming back if I keep coming to therapy. They (therapist or doctor) are so nice and knowledgeable, so there must be something wrong with me."

It's a fear-based business model—fear that there won't be another client, and fear that helping too quickly will create a scheduling void. But I've seen the opposite. *RoelsMethod*™ creates advocates. When you stop someone's pain in three sessions, they tell everyone. That one client becomes five. That one case becomes a reputation.

Our center is thriving—without gimmicks, without "hook and book" strategies, and without sacrificing integrity.

Other modalities often chase the pain. They concentrate the work on where the symptom shows up. They apply generic protocols and hope for the best. They work within familiar maps: upper traps for headaches, quadratus lumborum (QLs) for low back pain, and piriformis for sciatica. But what if the trap isn't the problem? What if the pain in the leg is a signal from a missed rotator?

RoelsMethod™ NeuroSomatic Intervention breaks those assumptions.

It teaches you to decode the body's compensations—to identify where the brain is guarding, where the real tension lives, and how to resolve it without force, guesswork, or extended dependency.

This isn't just a technique. It's a shift in thinking. And not everyone is ready.

But the clients are. They are exhausted, over-treated, under-heard, and desperate for results. *They don't care about your method—they care about their life.* They want to walk without wincing. Sleep without pills. Sit through dinner without shooting pain. Play with their kids. Work their job. Dance again. Laugh again.

They want what I wanted: their life back.

And that's what *RoelsMethod*™ gives them.

Chapter Three

What Makes RoelsMethod™ Different?

RoelsMethod™ NeuroSomatic Intervention stands alone because it was developed **outside** of the echo chamber of traditional rehab models—and that's precisely why it works.

I didn't invent this system in a lab. I invented it while trying to survive—and eventually solve—my debilitating pain. I've sat in the same treatment rooms, heard the same dismissive advice, and cried through the same nights. That experience didn't just make me empathetic. It made me **relentless**.

Other methods focus on managing pain. RoelsMethod™ is about *resetting* the neuromuscular system—not with guesswork, but with a protocol that locates the actual *muscle of origin.* Most people are shocked when I work on an area seemingly unrelated to their pain and the problem resolves instantly. That's the power of understanding the body's interconnected compensations.

Some key differences:

- **Rapid Relief**—Results are often felt in the first session, with a complete reset typically achieved in just three sessions.
- **Root-Cause Focused**—We don't treat the site of pain. We treat the source, often far removed from where the pain is felt.

- **Body and Brain Reset**—RoelsMethod™ unwinds the muscular confusion caused by injury, chronic stress, or overuse.
- **Clear Protocol**—A step-by-step method is in place. It's not energy work. It's not intuition-based. It's a system that can be learned.
- **Exclusive Access**—The RoelsMethod™ Pain Relief Center is the only place this method is practiced and taught. There is no franchise. No watered-down seminar. This is an elite, intimate, and practical experience.

And yes—I've taught in massage schools. I own two businesses. I offer more than

100 hours of nationally certified CE classes. But what truly sets this work apart is the *proof*.

Client after client has walked in skeptical and walked out stunned. Not because of hype, but because their pain was finally gone—after everything else failed.

RoelsMethod™ isn't about being the best therapist in the room. It's about being the last therapist they'll ever need.

Chapter Four
The Anatomy of a Reset

Pressure without precision is just force. Precision without breath is just anatomy.

Marry the two—and the nervous system listens.

1. Why Traditional Maps Fail

The overwhelming majority of musculoskeletal charts still label pain according to where it hurts. Low-back pain? Work the spinal erectors. Tension headache? Rub the upper traps. Sciatica? Stretch the piriformis. However, modern pain science literature tells a different story. In chronic cases, fewer *than 20 percent* of symptoms originate in the tissue that hurts; the rest stem from dysfunctional signaling higher up the neuromuscular chain, often two, three, or even four structures removed from the complaint.

RoelsMethod™ reverses the usual logic:

Conventional Approach		**RoelsMethod™ NeuroSomatic Intervention**
1. Find the pain.		1. Map the *compensation pattern.*
2. Treat where it hurts.		2. Reset the true instigator muscle.
3. Repeat weekly.		3. Confirm change immediately—often in minutes.

2. The Three-Point Map™

When a new client walks in, we gather three coordinates before ever laying hands:

> **Trajectory**—*When* did it first appear, and *where* has it migrated?
>
> **Trigger**—What **physical trauma** or **emotional stressor** showed up 3 to 6 months before onset?
>
> **Tolerance**—What single motion or posture brings it from a 3 to an 8?

Those answers narrow the field to a predictable shortlist of deep stabilizers (iliacus, SCM, diaphragm, soleus, etc.).

We test them with light palpation; the one that feels “weirdly sore—in a good way” is the problem muscle 95 percent of the time.

3. The Static-Breath Reset

- Sink two relaxed fingers into the belly of the muscle until the client reports a **3–5/10** tenderness.
- **Do not move.**
- Ask for **three slow, nasal inhales followed by open-mouth exhales.**
- **Maintain identical pressure**.
  At breath two or three, the tenderness melts. Nothing in your fingers changed. Everything in the client's *brain* did. That is the reset.

4. Layer, Confirm, Move On

- Two to three depths *maximum* in one muscle.
- Re-check the original symptomatic motion at the ten-minute mark.
- If the change is 60 percent or more, you're on the right track. If not, you're on the wrong muscle—adjust immediately; don't waste a session chasing the bad tissue.

5. Locking It In: Micro-Repatterning

A reset without reinforcement is a software patch that never saves. We teach **hourly 3-minute micro-stretches** that oppose the client's day-to-day posture. Even at 50 percent compliance, that's 25 30 minutes of corrective input per day—far beyond any once-a-week outpatient protocol.

6. Proof in Real Time

Most people leave the first visit stunned:

- The shoulder that couldn't abduct past 90° now reaches 160°.
- Migraine aura evaporates mid-table.
- The sciatic buzz that had haunted them for a year cycles down to zero before they stand up.

Not because we "fixed" tissue, but because we rewrote faulty code.

Key Take-away: *If the symptom hasn't dropped by at least half in 15 minutes, you're not on the right muscle. Be humble, pivot, and identify the actual cause.*

Chapter Five

Multiplying the Impact—
From Unicorn to Movement

I’m often called a unicorn. I accept it—but only as *proof of concept*. If one therapist can do this consistently, ten can, a hundred can, a thousand can. ***Chronic pain is a global crisis;*** we need an army of reset-artists.

1. The Reluctance of the Status-Quo

I’ve invited chiropractors and PTs to learn the work.

Their answer? “Why would I solve a case in three visits when I can sell thirty?”

That fear-based mindset is their ceiling, not mine. At the RoelsMethod™ Pain

Relief Center we stay **fully booked** not by locking clients into long plans, but by liberating them so quickly they tell *everyone* they know.

2. Nationally Certified Education

- **100+ hours of accredited CE** already produced.
- Technician-to-Educator track in development (see Appendix C).
- Training stays on-site—quality over quantity until we have a cadre who can replicate 90-percent first-visit change rates.

3. The RoelsMethod™ Support Circle

Relief is step one; staying free is step two. Weekly support circles blend gentle movement, guided breath work, and peer accountability. Members learn to

- Spot early warning signs of re-compensation.
- Use a 5-minute self-reset if needed.
- Share victories to reinforce neuroplastic change (community = dopamine = sustained habits).

4. A Call to Future Practitioners

If you're a therapist or healthcare worker reading this and you feel that familiar tug—equal parts curiosity and disbelief—know this:

- You will *work less hard* with your hands.
- You will see *faster transformations* than you've ever witnessed.
- You will, inevitably, shake your head and smile when a client whispers, "Why doesn't everyone do it this way?"

Because most people never get permission to believe healing can be that fast.

5. The Economics of Integrity

Helping in three sessions is not bad business; it's *excellent* business:

Model	Average Patient Value	Word-of-Mouth Multiplier	Reputation Curve
24-visit PT package	$2400	1–2 referrals (fatigue) @ $2,400 – $4,800	Flat
3-visit Roels reset	$750	5–8 referrals (awe) @ $3,750–$6,000	Exponential
Do the math: solving problems scales *better* than prolonging them. (And it's easier on your own body and administrative overhead)			

6. Next Steps

- **For Clients:** Finish the 30-day Reset Workbook, then share your result online using @RoelsMethodReset. Your story is someone else's lifeline.
- **For Therapists:** Apply for the next Technician Cohort. Expect to unlearn half of what school taught you—and to fall back in love with why you entered this field.
- **For Skeptics:** Book a session. Bring your toughest, longest-standing pain. Most people are no longer skeptical at the end of that session.

Purpose, not ego, drives this work. I'm not better than anyone—I'm unwilling to let outdated models profit from preventable suffering.

Chapter Six

The 30-Day NeuroSomatic Reset Blueprint

Give the nervous system 30 days of clear signals, and it will write you an entirely new owner's manual.

1. Why Thirty Days?

- **Neuroplasticity research** shows that consistent, *daily* input over 4-to-5 weeks lays down new synaptic wiring.
- **Chronic-pain MRI studies** reveal measurable decreases in limbic-system reactivity after **21-to-30 days** of breath-based somatic practice.

Thirty days isn't random—it's biology.

2. The Macro Arc

(Week by Week Overview)

Week	Primary Objective	Daily Time-Ask
1	*Interrupt the Threat Loop*—static-breath resets for 2 to 3 core instigators.	15 min
2	*Re-ignite Prime Mover*—micro-stretches that oppose your baseline posture.	18 min
3	*Wire in Safety*—add diaphragmatic breath + 5-min visualization.	23 min
4	*Stress-Proof the Pattern*—movement, snacks + community share.	25 min

3. Daily Skeleton

~**Morning Check-In** 90 seconds

- Scan body, rate symptom on a scale of 0–10, and jot it in the log.
- **Static-Breath Reset**—3 minutes Pick one instigator muscle (iliacus, SCM, soleus, etc.). Two fingers, 3 breaths.
- **Micro-Stretch**—3 minutes Counter-posture from your work life (pec corner stretch if you desk-sit; hip-flexor lunge if you drive).

~Five-Minute Visualization

(Weeks 3–4)

Eyes closed. See yourself moving, working, laughing pain-free. Anchor the feeling, not just the image.

~Evening Debrief—90 seconds

Re-score symptoms. Note *what improved and when.* Pattern-tracking beats guesswork.

4. The Non-Negotiables

- **Hourly Movement Alarm**—200 steps or one full micro-stretch circuit.
- **Hydration**—drink a minimum half your body-weight in ounces; fascia without water is Velcro.
- **Sleep Target**—7+ hours; growth hormone bursts at night help finish the muscular remodel.

5. Troubleshooting Guide

Road Block	Likely Cause	Fix
Pain spikes after reset	Too much pressure	Back off 30 percent; redo breaths
Head feels “floaty”	Hyper-ventilating	Slow inhale to 4-count, exhale to 6.
Motivation tanks at Day 12	Dopamine dip (normal)	Text a Reset-Buddy a 20-sec video update. Accountability = neurotransmitter boost

6. Graduating Day 30

By now, you should have experienced:

- **85-to-90 percent** symptom reduction.
- A library of *self-led resets* you can deploy in under five minutes.
- Proof—written in your log—that your body is *trainable*, not broken.

Remember: *When something flares in the future, you're not starting over—you're swinging a tool you already own.*

Chapter Seven: Your Ecosystem of Ongoing Freedom

"Healing that stays private is a candle under a basket—bright, but wasting its power."

1. The Support-Circle Model

Every Thursday evening at the RoelsMethod™ Pain Relief Center, clients meet in a semi-circle of mats and chairs:

- Three-minute diaphragmatic breathing.
- A single round-robin question: *"What changed this week?"*
- A 15-minute guided mobility flow.
- Open Q&A with a Certified RoelsMethod™ Technician.

Data point: Members who attend at least **two circles per month** report an additional **21 percent decline** in pain recurrence at the six-month follow-up.

2. Recruiting Your "Sounding Board" of Directors

- **Movement Ally**—workout buddy, stretch partner, or dog demanding daily walks.
- **Nervous-System Ally**—a therapist, coach, or mentor who reminds you to *breathe before you react*.
- **Reality-Check Ally**—someone who will lovingly call BS when you slip back into martyr stories.

Three humans. Zero apps required.

3. When to Book a Tune-Up

- A familiar twinge jumps more than **3-points** on your 0-10 scale and lingers for 48 hours.
- You nail a major fitness PR or finish a race—*celebrate with a reset*, not just beer and selfies.
- Life drops a stress bomb (loss, move, breakup). Emotional load changes muscle firing—catch it early.

4. Integrating With (or despite) the Medical System

Bring your prescription list, your MRI, and your post-op notes—fine.
What you won't bring is the hidden assumption that tissues heal in straight lines or on insurance-dictated timelines.
RoelsMethod™ mantra: *We collaborate when medicine helps, and we pioneer when medicine shrugs.*

5. Spreading the Fire

- Share your Before/After story on social media with #RoelsMethodReset.
- Give a copy of this book to one person still trapped in the revolving-door model.
- Invite your PT, chiropractor, or yoga teacher to the *Intro to NeuroSomatic Logic* workshop. If they decline? Your conscience is clear—you offered a lifeline.

6. For Therapists Ready to Jump

- **Technician Cohort Applications** open quarterly.
- Prereqs: existing license, anatomy fluency, willingness to unlearn dogma.
- Expect 24 hours of live drill, 30 logged resets, and a 90-percent first-visit success threshold before certification.
  If you need twelve sessions to prove you're effective, that's okay—*it just isn't RoelsMethod*™.

7. Closing Charge

You now possess knowledge that dismantles decades of "just-manage-it" despair. Whether you're a client who finally moved without flinching or a practitioner who watched a migraine vanish under your fingertips, the opportunity and responsibility is the same:

Keep the circle widening.

Pain relieved in one body is a victory; pain relieved in a community is a revolution.

Chapter 8:

Why We Built a Circle, Not a Waiting Room

The RoelsMethod™ Support Circle—Healing in Community

"Pain shared is pain divided; hope shared is hope multiplied."

For years, I watched clients walk out of treatment rooms lighter in body yet still carrying the emotional weight of chronic pain: frustration, isolation, and the subtle shame that says, *"Why hasn't my body healed yet?"* Traditional clinics send those feelings back home with a print-out of stretches and a reminder card.

RoelsMethod™ takes a different view: the nervous system is a social organ. Safety, co-regulation, and witnessed progress accelerate neurosomatic change. That is why every new client is automatically invited into the **Support Circle**—a lightly facilitated small-group gathering that meets once a week for the first month of care and once a month thereafter.

8.1 How the Circle Works

Element	Purpose	Neuroscience Hook
Check-In Round (5 min each)	Verbalize wins, challenges, fears	Naming emotion moves activity from limbic system → prefrontal cortex, reducing threat signaling
Guided Breath Reset (3 min)	Group coherence and vagal tone	Synchronized exhale lengthens heart-rate variability, calming sympathetic drive
Mini-Lesson (10 min)	One bite-sized concept: central sensitization, compensation chains, etc.	Understanding lowers "fear-avoidance" behaviors linked to persistent pain
Partner Stretch or Self-Palpation Drill (7 min)	Embody the lesson	Kinesthetic learning cements new motor maps
Hope Share (closing)	30-second statement of what life looks like pain-free	Future visualization recruits default-mode network, boosting neuroplasticity

Circle size is capped at **10,** so everyone is seen. When enrollment exceeds capacity, we spin up another pod—it's fractal growth by design.

8.2 Outcomes We Track

- Over 90% average reduction in Pain Catastrophizing Scale after three treatments
- The referral rate from Circle members is 2.4 times higher than that of one-to-one clients, because people talk about a life-changing community, not just a clever technique.

8.3 Facilitation Guide for Practitioners

- **Hold the frame**—You're not coaching trauma stories; you're stewarding safety. Redirect ruminations back to the body.
- **Stay protocol-aligned**—Circle time is not a replacement for one-on-one clinical resets. It's the glue.
- **Model neutrality**—Celebrate wins without ego; honor struggles without rescue.
- **End on uplift**—Neuroplasticity favors the emotional tone that concludes the experience.

Client Voice

The sessions fixed my hip, but the Circle fixed my mindset. I stopped thinking of myself as "the broken one" and started cheering other people's progress. Somehow that made mine stick."

~Rosa L., 48, teacher

Chapter 9

Multiplying Impact—Training the Next Generation of NeuroSomatic Practitioners**

A method that stays in one pair of hands is a hobby.

A method that spreads responsibly becomes a movement.

The Bottleneck Problem

I spent my first decade in practice performing miracle-feeling resets, only to realize the math:

One therapist × five clients a day × 4 days a week = 1,000 lives a year.

That's beautiful—and wholly inadequate for the **50 million** Americans living with chronic musculoskeletal pain today. Scaling RoelsMethod™ required a training architecture as rigorous as the protocol itself.

9.1 Credential Pathway (2025 Edition)

The NCBTMB approves coursework; graduates will be nationally certified to teach over 100 hours of continuing education.

9.2 Why Some Professionals Push Back

"If RoelsMethod™ fixes people in three sessions, I'd have to find new patients every month."

~Unnamed chiropractor, 2021

Fear-based business models rely on symptom management rather than resolution. Our answer is simple economics:

- A complete-body reset commands **premium pricing**—clients happily pay for definitive results.
- Transformative outcomes drive **net-promoter word-of-mouth**

that fills schedules without sleight-of-hand retention tactics.

- **Diversified revenue**—workshops, retreat intensives, and digital follow-ups—keeps calendars full while honoring rapid relief.

9.3 Apprenticeship Inside the Pain Relief Center

New hires shadow three complete client arcs (initial + 2 follow-ups) before laying hands independently. Metrics for release:

- **90%+ accuracy** in identifying the prime mover on blind assessment.
- **Consistent 2-point drop** on client-reported pain scale within the first 15 minutes.
- **Clear, confident language** that explains the difference between reset and release without using jargon.

Those who pass are invited onto the floor and immediately integrated into the Support Circle schedule. Teaching reinforces mastery; within weeks, they're leading the mini-lesson segment for their pod.

9.4 Joining the Movement—An Invitation

If you're a therapist who's tired of twelve-minute muscle rubs and care plans that feel like hamster wheels, consider this your call to purpose. RoelsMethod™ doesn't ask you to work harder; it trains you to work *truer*—at the level where the nervous system makes decisions.

Three-session transformations are not detrimental to business; they are the best marketing strategy on earth.

The only question is whether you want to be part of a profession that measures success by the number of lives liberated, not the number of appointments booked.

"Healing shouldn't be a subscription model. Teach me to fish, and I'll feed a village."

~Michael Roels

Made in the USA
Columbia, SC
31 August 2025